The Lazy Man's

Guide

To Managing

Type 2 Diabetes

By Leslie R. Auger

Table of Contents

Introduction

I was numb. The impact of the Doctors words hadn't hit yet.
"You have Diabetes,..." he said.

Hi all. I want to introduce myself, My name is Leslie Auger and I am a type 2 diabetic. I will be sharing with you a brief account of my experience with managing this disease in the hopes that you will not be in the dark as long as I was..

I am not a Doctor, a nutritionist, or any other health worker. I am a regular guy who was diagnosed with type 2 diabetes back in 2000 during a regular health exam for my Commercial Drivers License, I am a truck driver.

I decided to write this short book because it wasn't until 2011 that I found a "cure" for my disease, largely because most of the information I was getting was coming from the medical profession which was confusing and often couched in medical-ease which quite honestly took me some time to sort through.

There really is no "cure" for diabetes, type 2 or type 1, once diagnosed with it you have it period.

That having been said there are ways in which you can manage the disease to slow down or even stop the damage that is occurring in your body from the excessive "sugar" flowing through your blood stream.

We all need this "sugar" it is the source of energy and and gives our body the ability to function, but too much of it damages our body just like too much electricity through your TV set will burn it out.

Our bodies have a built in regulator of sorts that preforms many functions, it's called the pancreas and it produces the insulin that delivers energy called glucose to your cells. .

When an electrical regulator is stressed too long or too often or is physically damaged it becomes a danger to the electrical systems it protects.

Type 2 diabetes is somewhat like that. The pancreas may have become stressed by infection and some of the cells died. These cells are unable to be replaced and they are the ones that manufacturer insulin.

The other cause that I am aware of (and is the focus of this book) is insulin resistance. Science does not yet know why, but for some reason insulin is prevented from delivering it's payload of glucose to our cells leaving too much glucose (sugar) in our blood.

Drug therapy is a great bandage, a temporary solution, but this disease is progressive meaning it will get worse over time requiring more and stronger drugs if the root cause is not dealt with.

I called this book the Lazy Man's Guide To

Managing Type 2 Diabetes because my method of management is simple by comparison and honestly I don't like to work that hard. Plus, I have done most of the hard work for you--- sorting through all the medical mumbo jumbo.

Well, on to my story so you can see I am not full of it.

My Story

Hi all, my name is Leslie Auger, I go by Les. At, the time of this writing (2015) I am a 56 year old male. I am also a truck driver which means that I have to undergo a physical at least every two years to keep my drivers licence. And that is how my diabetes was discovered.

Let me back up just a little bit, In the fall of 1999, I had had a few incidents that caused some property damage. Then I had one Friday night when I was headed home from Los Angeles, California, I pulled into a rest stop to get some sleep before finishing my trip. I woke up Sunday afternoon in a puddle of sweat. Something was wrong. My employer put me on medical leave until we could find out what the problem was.

Several months later all the bad news had come in. I had a tear in my retina, an abdominal hernia and diabetes.

I had gone in and given blood for testing, and few days later the lab called and said, "Mr Auger we need you to come back in and give more blood. I asked ,"why" they said, " something was wrong but we can't tell you until we are sure." I was worried to say the least, blood is the major highway that delivers all the nutrients and removes some of the waste that our bodies produce. My first thought was cancer.

Nearly a week later I was sitting in a Dr.'s office waiting to find out what the problem was.

The Dr. popped his head in and in lest than 2 minuets delivered the bad news," You have Diabetes, here is a few pamphlets, I teach a class on Thursdays." and out the door he went. Later I found out that the reason the lab called me back in was that they couldn't believe the test results since I was on my feet and basically feeling fine. They thought they had made an error, My blood glucose level was over 600 mg/dl.

The pamphlets the Dr. had given me were worthless, they told me nothing about this disease and even less about managing it. I didn't like this Dr. and his manner so I began to look for another and soon found a Doctor by the name of Zimmet. He was an unusual Doctor in that he was a regular physician, a naturopath and a psychologist, a very brilliant man. I was very lucky because he rarely took in new patients but just happened to have an opening when I called.

Dr. Z. took the time to explain in laymen terms what the disease is. He began me on a regiment of Metformian and recommended that I get the book "Protein Power" by Dr. and Dr. Eades and read it before I came back the following week.

I got the book and read it from cover to cover in just a few days. Wow, what a powerful book, (and some great recipes too). On my next visit Dr. Z told me that I could manage this disease through diet, **IF**, I followed the diet suggested in the book. He said that in just a few months, doing the diet, I could get off the pills. He was right.

I did have one of the side effects of Metformian, diarrhea, explosive diarrhea. Dr. Z said to stay on it for another week or two while my body adjusted to it. It didn't and it made no difference to my blood sugar so we switched to Glipizide, it did work. I followed the diet and three months later I was off the drug.

The protein diet worked well for about three years, but I paid no attention to volume, after all, the book said I could eat all the lean meat I wanted (I ignored the lean part of lean meat) and all the mayonnaise I wanted. I went hog wild and kept gaining weight.

I had been about 260 lbs at 5'8" when I was diagnosed and as a truck driver combined, with the fact that I resent "exercise", I just kept gaining weight and of course my blood sugar readings kept rising.

Not all type 2 diabetics are overweight but the vast majority of us are.

Dr. Z retired and I was unable to find a Dr. anywhere near as wise or intelligent as he. I floundered around from doctor to doctor for the next eight years. Both my weight and blood sugar kept going up. I was put back on pills. Then a combination of pills, then Byeta, which is a none insulin injectable, (more on drugs later). Truck drivers who use insulin are disqualified from working until they can prove they can use the drug without the side effect of low blood sugar, so I was trying everything I could to avoid being put on insulin.

Finally, in 2009, my Doctor said there is nothing more that can be done and I had to go on Insulin. My A1c was a whopping 13.6.

By then I was weighing 350 lbs or better and my blood sugar was averaging about 260 with the drugs.

I was refereed to an endocrinologist. I was devastated, my career was over, I had no way to earn a living that would keep my family at the comfort level they had become accustomed to.

I had asked the endocrinologist if he had ever seen anyone get off insulin once they were put on it. He said "No". In my heart I said "watch me". Don't know where that came from, I think it was my God.

About 10 months later I was introduced to a way of eating that was more balanced and focused on quantity as well as quality. I adopted this way of eating and within 6 months I had dropped about 80 lbs and was off all medication. That was in 2011 and I have been off all drugs since that time, I had gotten my A1c down to 5.8.

At the time of this writing I have gained back some weight because I got sloppy with the diet so my last A1c was 6.4 still acceptable but a clear warning.

Well that's my story. It's still unfolding and I am learning more all the time, but as you can see the only credential I have is I have diabetes and so far am winning the battle.

What is Diabetes?

I will attempt to answer this question as simply as I can. That being said I am not a doctor or a researcher and there is new information coming out all the time. This is my understanding after reading many websites and books.

There are two classes of diabetes, Type 1 and Type 2.

Type 1 is simply that the pancreas is not producing sufficient insulin. This is an immediate life threatening disease and without insulin the person will die, it is usually discovered in childhood.

Type 2 diabetes (also known as diabetes mellitus) is much more complicated and in my opinion is actually miss-classified. Some researchers prefer the term Insulin Resistance Syndrome, which is more accurate but still does not cover all the variations in the illness.

The majority of us that suffer from this disease have the insulin resistant type. What that means is your pancreas is producing insulin but for some reason not yet understood it is not able to preform it's job.

What is insulin's Job?

Well for starters insulin is a hormone that is created in the pancreas to make and transfer glucose to your body's cells. It acts much like a gasoline pump, delivering fuel to your car. Insulin will also turn excess glucose into fat for later use and convert that fat back to glucose as needed. This is a simplistic explanation and this hormone does more jobs than this but, it's primary job is delivering fuel to your body's cells.

It does it's job by converting the carbohydrates (flour, vegetables, sugars) that we eat into a substance known as glucose and then delivering the glucose to our cells. In the insulin resistance form of type 2 diabetes, the glucose is prevented from being delivered to the cells. This condition can seriously affect how you feel and function and will eventually lead to serious health issues. Untreated, it will cause a slow and painful death.

This condition is progressive. Untreated it gets worse, treated by medication helps but does not stop the underlying cause. Diet modification significantly slows the progression and can actually save you from a slow and painful death.

What can happen to you if you decided not to treat your diabetes?

Heart disease, Vascular disease, Blindness, Kidney disease, Gum disease, damage to your nerves leading to loss of sensation or pain and even stomach and bowel problems.

A disease that leads to sure and quick death is much easier to face than to face disease that will slowly torture you to death.

Still thinking about not making those simple changes in your lifestyle to control this disease? If you are than consider volunteering to be a prisoner of terrorist group, it would be an easier and faster death.

Drug Therapy

I want to talk about drug therapy because this is the Doctors first line of defence against this disease and while it is a good first step, it needs to be just that, a first step. All too often, it is the only step.

Drugs help but, they are a bandage on an infected cut where a good cleansing and stitches are needed.

If you read my story then you know that the drugs helped to a point, once I crossed that invisible line the drugs where no longer effective. The reason is simple the underlying cause of the disease was not being treated.

Remember that insulin has a job to perform and in type 2 diabetes it is being prevented from doing it for some unknown reason. Insulin is not delivering the life sustaining fuel to the cells. Increasing insulin creation, which is what most drugs do, will not improve this condition.

There are many Drugs used in the treatment of type 2 diabetes and for the scope of this book I have decided not to include a list but instead to refer you to a web site.

http://www.diabetes.org/living-with-diabetes/treatment-and-care/medication/oral-medications/what-are-my-options.html

It's a long link but the information is worth

checking out.

Make sure that if you are taking other drugs that both your doctor and your pharmacist know what those are. Ask if there are any known interactions with any drug you may already be taking, over the counter or prescription.

I repeat drugs are a good first step, but please, don't let it be your only step. You can live a long and productive life with this disease if you make a few simple lifestyle changes.

As a final note, please be aware that most oral medications have the side effect of weight gain. This is one of the main reasons why diet is a much better option since being overweight contributes to the disease more than any other normal factor, but your doctor **_MUST_** be the final judge as to weather or not you need to be on a drug.

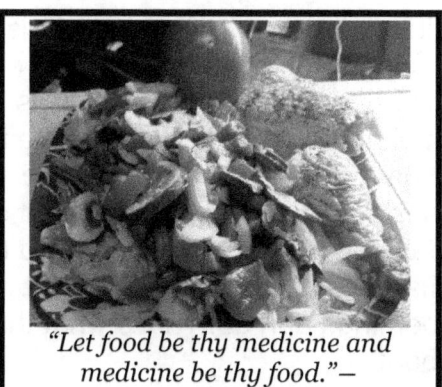

"Let food be thy medicine and medicine be thy food."—
Hippocrates

How I Manage My Diabetes

There are some really great resources for the person willing to spend the time reading through the massive amounts of information out there, especially on the internet. The American Diabetes Association (ADA) is a great place to start.

Throughout all of the resources you will find three basic fundamentals:

A. eat right
B. sleep right
C. and get exercise

There are two more common factors mentioned in nearly all the literature, they are

a. quit smoking
b. quit caffeinated drinks

With me being a truck driver, C. is out of the question, just isn't going to happen (not to mention my resentment against it). B. isn't going to happen either, and while I would love to quit smoking I haven't been able to yet. And, as far as caffeinated drinks go, well, does a habit of a half gallon a day of coffee sound like I could quit, nope that ain't happening either. But eat right, now that's something I can do. That's what this little book is about.

There is an old saying, "you are what you eat", like it or not it is true. Another saying I have heard is "if you eat well, you will be well"' I believe it! It has worked for me!

Okay, so here are the basics:

Breakfast
      1 Citrus fruit
      1/2 cup of Oatmeal
      6 ounces of a lean protein

Lunch
      2 cups green salad mix
      1 cup green vegetable
      1 apple
      6 ounces of lean protein

Dinner
      Repeat the lunch

2 snacks are allowed if needed and should be 3 ounces of a _lean_ protein or a piece of fruit.

Ladies, you do not need as much protein

as a man so modify this by making your protein portion 4 ounces instead of 6 ounces.

Beyond the Basics.

I have learned that it takes between 4 to 6 hours for our stomachs to process the food we eat, so, as a rule of thumb I keep my meals spaced by at least that amount. I do not like to go beyond 6 hours because I get too hungry and the meal does not satisfy. If it is necessary to space a meal beyond 6 hours I will use a snack.

Breakfast, is always within the first hour after rising (my schedule can vary significantly from day to day). It does not matter if I am hungry or not, breakfast stimulates our metabolism out of the slower sleep mode and will get our minds and bodies functioning better for the day.

Eating on a schedule is important because our bodies need a steady flow of nutrients and calories. Getting hungry is the early warning signal that the fuel tank is nearly empty.

Snacking through out the day as some of us do does not allow our bodies to function as they were designed to function and can confuse the insulin production and the efficiency of our digestive tract.

Some dietitians will not like my food plan because it does not include dairy. Milk is made for baby cows, not humans and there is a large body of evidence that cow milk harms the human system. I don't like saying that because my income is made from the sale of milk, but it is true. If you must have dairy, use it sparingly, Yogourt (without added sugar) is the best source of dairy.

If Calcium is your concern, green vegetables will more than meet your calcium needs unless you have a deficiency caused by disease.

While I still consume massive amounts of coffee, I would never consider soda pop not even diet. Processed sugar is okay in small amounts, *very small amounts*, our bodies do not process it well. And, the committee is still out on artificial sweeteners. I have a friend whose primary interest was loosing weight, he only did one thing and that was to stop drinking soda pop and lost up to five pounds a week until he stabilized some 25 pounds lighter. Besides all that I just don't like the after taste or the wasting of my calorie count on useless calories.

Talking about calories, if you do not add any calories with dressing, sauces or whatever, this food plan runs about 1800 to1900 calories per day for men and about 1500 to 1600 calories for women which is optimal for loosing about 3 pounds a week if your sedentary like I am. If you move your body more than a truck driver does then you may need a bit more. There are charts to help you determine this.

Because of the food production practises in this and other countries have become dependent on artificial means of nutrients for the plants, it is necessary to supplement with artificial vitamins and minerals.

I use a multi-vitamin, B complex, 2000, milligrams of Cinnamon and 2000 milligrams of Fish Oil per day.

I also use a heaping tablespoon of Cinnamon to season my oatmeal with. Cinnamon does help with sugar control. I do not use sweeteners on my oatmeal. It did take a few days to get use to no sweeter but now I prefer it

It really doesn't matter what proteins you use except that it *must be lean*. Devoid of fat as much as possible. If you use eggs I recommend you boil them, don't fry them in oil, period.

Don't eat fried foods, those are guaranteed to raise your blood sugar as well as your cholesterol and triglycerides, plus they are very high in calories.

I know, it sounds like a boring way to eat but would you rather have the excitement of being blind or maybe the emotional rush of preparing for an amputation or maybe the drama of a heart attack is more your style. It's really your choice.

Forget about pastries and flour products. Besides who wants to eat paste (remember grade school making paste with flour and water). Flour is so processed that it no longer adequately represents the seed it came from, holds no nutritional value to speak of except calories.

Yes, flour products raise blood sugar.

Once you get control of your blood sugar then you can splurge once in a while and have a piece of pizza or a doughnut but for now just stick to the food plan.

Oh, ya, once in a while is not every other day, your body has to have time to recovery from the abuse, just like it does from a black eye or a cut.

So, you have decided to try this way of eating for a time, what can you expect.

I will share with you my experience which seems to be fairly representative of all the people I have talked to that have tried this or similar food plans.

The first three days or so I experienced hunger between meals but then suddenly I found myself rarely keeping my schedule because I just wasn't hungry If I moved more than usual then I would need to use my snacks.

It took about three weeks before I began to notice any weight loss, but once it started it was consistent.

I can not remember exactly when it was that my blood sugar began to drop but it seemed it was about the same time I began noticing the weight coming off.

One more change will be your bowels.

This is a good thing. I had been suffering from hemorrhoids they stopped being a problem.

Expect more gas for the first few months, annoying, but it will normalize in time.

I began this food plan February, 11 of 2011 and it was July, 9th of 2011 that my endocrinologist took me off insulin one more week and I was taken off the pills.

Testing your blood glucose level during this time is critical, especially if you are on any type of diabetic drugs. Low blood sugar can be more dangerous than high blood sugar and is easier to correct. Low blood sugar can cause you to pass out and go into a comma if not corrected quickly.

Should you begin to feel faint or weak immediately check your blood sugar level if it's too low take some glucose tablets or eat an orange or drink orange juice. Then call your doctor. Your medication dose may need to be adjusted.

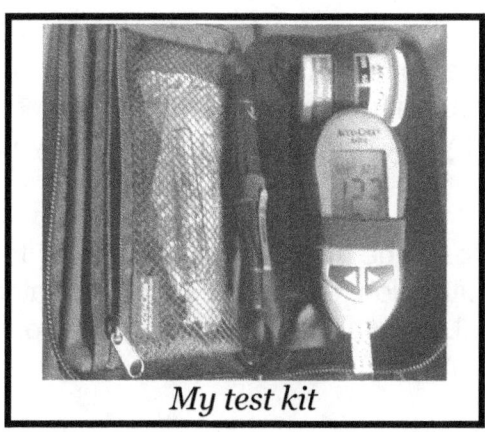
My test kit

Testing, When, How, and Why

For this chapter I am going to assume you are newly diagnosed.

I will state again that I am not a doctor and all I am doing is sharing my experience with you. I have been dealing with this disease for fifteen years, the last three years I can claim success in the reversal of this disease. But that does not make me an expert. The expert is your doctor. Listen to what he/she says then DO IT.

Your doctor is your best friend in dealing with this disease and if he/she knows you are following their advice they will be more inclined to go the extra mile to help you. They get so many patients that will not follow what they advise that after a while they get a bit calloused, I think you can understand that.

Be considerate of your Doctors time and make notes of anything you wish to ask about before your meetings with him/her. The notes will also help you to be more clear on what you want to know.

Do not be afraid to bring anything to you doctors attention, even if it seems unrelated to the disease. Like I said earlier, insulin is a hormone that has many functions in the body.

There are the rare Doctors out there that are in it just for the money, but most are not and if you show a real desire to manage your disease your doctor will perk up and be of real service to you. But if you are seeing a Doc that doesn't really care, fire him/her, like, yesterday. They work for you, you pay their bills.

So lets talk about your other new friend called the glucose meter.

Yes, you will need one, they can be cheap or expensive depending on how many bells and whistles you want, truthfully though all you really need is one that will give you an accurate reading and keep in memory your averages . For the last two years I have been using the Accu-Chek by Aviva. I am very satisfied with it.

You do not need a prescription to buy a meter or it's test strips unless you want your insurance to pay for it. The test strips are a one shot item and that is where the cost is. Each test will cost you between 75 cents to a dollar and a half or more. I test three times a day and will explain why in a minute. Most insurances will pay most of the cost of the strips provided you get the meter they want you to have.

I will not go into the test procedure as the instructions in the box are usually very easy to understand.

Using the glucose meter is one of two tests that you will be doing on a regular basis. The other test is the A1c test which is usually done by your doctors office every three to six months. This test is done by drawing blood and sending it to a lab. There is a meter that you can buy that will preform this test at home but it is expensive and I have not looked into it, some doctors offices use it.

Why use the blood glucose meter?

The simplest reason is to see if your management program is working. The meter checks your blood sugar level in the here and now and can show you in real time what effect different foods have on your blood sugar.

If your management program is working as well as my plan has worked for me, the meter can save your bacon, especially if your feeling a bit odd and don't know why. Without the meter you may not know you are crashing (blood sugar dropping too low) until it's too late.

The A1c test shows an average over approximately 3 months and is of a great use to see what the over all effect of your management program has been. Plus it will tell the Doctor if you have been lying to him/her about the management of your disease.

I said I test three times a day, the reason is because I want to know what certain foods do to my blood sugar. Most insurance will not pay for testing that often unless you are on insulin. I get mine thru the VA and pay about 25 dollars for three months worth of strips. My doctor was willing to write this script because she has seen how I manage my disease.

My Doc has seen how I manage my disease because I keep good records. I record every reading on a graph that I developed and is shown in the photo at the end of this chapter.

My records show my meter reading and the time of day that I took it. I also record everything that I have ate and at what time of day I ate it, even if it is something I knew I should not have ate. I even record any exercise and excessive emotional times (anger, fear, stress, etc.) I may have had that day no matter how trivial it may have been.

Record keeping is important to keep you honest with yourself and help your doctor to help you.

So what "test" numbers are we looking for. Well your Doctor will inform you as to when and how often he/she wants you to test and they should tell you what "target range" they want to see. But the following chart is a good general rule of thumb.

Before a meal	70–130 mg/dl
1-2 hours after beginning of a meal	Less than 180 mg/dl

These numbers are your goals and will tell you that your glucose is under control if they are consistently in these ranges. If they are not then changes may need to be made. Consult you doctor before making any changes.

If the numbers are in the 70's consistently get on the phone and ask your doctor what to do. Below 70 and you could be in a crises and should seek medical help immediately. I personally begin to feel faint when I hit 77 and immediately reach for an orange which was what my doctor has recommended.

Here is a chart to help you determine what your A1c test results mean:

A1C level	Estimated average blood sugar level
5 percent	97 mg/dL (5.4 mmol/L)
6 percent	126 mg/dL (7 mmol/L)
7 percent	154 mg/dL (8.5 mmol/L)
8	183 mg/dL (10.2 mmol/L)

percent	
9 percent	212 mg/dL (11.8 mmol/L)
10 percent	240 mg/dL (13.3 mmol/L)
11 percent	269 mg/dL (14.9 mmol/L)
12 percent	298 mg/dL (16.5 mmol/L)
13 percent	326 mg/dL (18.1 mmol/L)
14 percent	355 mg/dL (19.7 mmol/L)

From:http://www.mayoclinic.org/tests-procedures/a1c-test/basics/results/prc-20012585

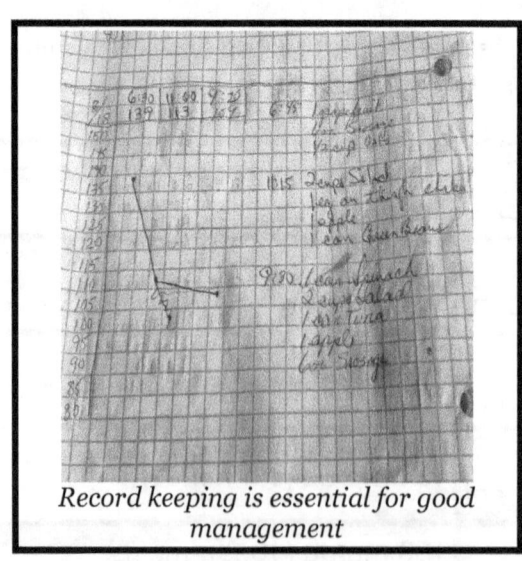

Record keeping is essential for good management

Exercise

I don't, plain and simple.

The most exercise I get is going from the back of the parking lot at a truck stop to the rest room. Most days I don't have the time but when I do, I don't because I hate anything resembling exercise and have ever since that load mouthed Drill Sargent in basic training, I hate that guy!

In my research I have found that exercise does work to lower blood sugar.

The few times I have taken a long walk my B/S numbers did improve for about 24 hours. So if you don't hate it then add it to your management plan.

This is another one of those items you need to ask your doctor about. He/she knows your physical condition and if they don't have knowledge about what is appropriate for you they will be able to direct you to someone who does.

If you want to do it, and can do it, then do it.

As a means of burning calories, exercise is highly overrated. Simply put you can not work off the calories of a day of indulgence by an hour at the gym,.But, as a means of improving your metabolism and hence your blood sugar, it is the ticket, provided you do it regularly.

One of my dearest friends is a Ti Chi

instructor which is a very mild form of exercise and at 77 years old she has the body of a twenty year old. And, too old to start is bunk, she started in her sixties. Of further note she does teach handicapped and other elderly folk so the bottom line is if you want to, there is an exercise program out there for you.

If you do decide to exercise and especially if you are on meds keep very close eye on your blood sugar numbers, you may have to decrease your dose of medication and /or increase your calories. But, as always let your doctor be the final judge of any changes in your management program.

Uncontrolled Diabetes

Okay, so you have decided that making the few changes it takes to manage your diabetes is just too much like work. You will just take the medicine and eat what you want when you want.

Fine, it's your choice, but, I want you to be aware of the consequences of your choice.

Drugs help but they are not the solution.

Remember I had said that at the time I was diagnosed they had also found tears in my retina. It happened again only much more seriously within this past year. I have no doubt I would be blind by now if I hadn't gotten control of this disease when I did.

I have had some nerve damage as well causing a loss of sensation in my hands which makes it difficult to sense small objects.

I also had to have cataract surgery at the young age of 53, also diabetic related.

Of further note, is sexual function and while age has played a part in it I am equally sure that the diabetes has played a much bigger part in my lack of response to my wife, the desire is there but the body doesn't respond.

All of these reasons are why I decided to put this little book together. This disease can affect every organ in your body *and it will if left* _untreated._ So, do yourself a favour and get on the wagon. The better the control you have of this disease will result in minimizing or even stalling the damage it does.

I will again repeat that drug therapy is a good start but if you do not deal with this disease at it's roots, meaning lifestyle and the foods you eat, it will continue it's progression.

Here is a list of all the 'conditions' untreated diabetes can cause:

1. Heart and blood-vessel disease: coronary-artery disease, heart attack, stroke, narrowing of arteries, and high blood pressure

2.Nerve damage (neuropathy): tingling, numbness, burning or pain of the toes or fingers

3.Kidney damage (nephropathy)

4.Eye damage (diabetic retinopathy)

5.Poor blood flow and circulation to the feet resulting in various complications including amputation.

6.Increased susceptibility to skin infections or poor healing of wounds

7. Gum disease and infection

If eating the cake or candy with it's momentary sense of pleasure is worth living day in and day out with the pain and discomfort these complications will cause, then have at it, enjoy while you can.

Getting Help

This little book is designed primarily as a "primer". There is tons of more information out there to help you and your doctor design and implement a management program that will work for you.

If you are interested in more information to managing your disease I recommend several websites to begin your education with.

The first is the American Diabetes Association, their website is:

http://www.diabetes.org/

Another great resource is Joslin Diabetes Centre:

http://www.joslin.org/index.html

These few are just a place to begin your research.

You may find that changing you eating habits is incredibly difficult. There are many organizations out there that offer support groups. I use one but they wish to be anonymous so I wont be able to tell you who they are. However, look and you will find. Many are free.

All this being said your doctor should be your number one resource.

Another great professional resource is a Nutritionist. Most have knowledge that doctors do not have as far as how food works in your system. Many doctors will refer you to a Nutritionist, if yours does, then use them.

If your doctor does not refer you to a nutritionist then check out this web site to find one near you:

http://www.eatright.org/find-an-expert

For my Trucker Friends

You know that living on the road is not a healthy way to live. We sit in the drivers seat 10 to 14 hours a day then move to the bunk for 10 hours then back to the seat. It's hard on every bit of our body.

It is not uncommon for health issues to end our career before we are of the age to qualify for Medicare or any other State medical help.

As I found out the hard way, if you are put on insulin you can not work until you can prove to the Federal Government that you can use insulin safely, meaning you don't pass out behind the wheel from low blood sugar. To do this will require about ten months during which you will not be making an income and will have to pay an Endocrinologist and a General MD every three months, plus the cost of insulin and test strips.

Once the wavier is received you will be able to go back to work but will have to continue to see the Endocrinologist and send in reports to the FMCSA. Your medical card will be restricted to one year and may even be valid for less time than that depending on your doctors evaluation of your management program.

Today, using my food plan, as outlined in this book I take no drugs whatever except over the counter vitamins and a prescription level of potassium due to an unrelated heart issue.

My food plan can be used in the truck. I have found foods that I can store in my ice chest, that are precooked and provide the necessary nutrition. Commercially bagged salad mix stays fresh for a week as long as you keep ice on it.

Wall Mart Supper Centre's have everything I need and as you know they are one of the few markets that allow us to park in their lot.

There is a ton of information on the internet that is geared for us, by us, so put your lap top, notebook or phone to good use while waiting on loads and get informed. But most importantly DO IT! Manage this disease! It's you life and your livelihood.

I do have a blog which I don't write on much but does contain some more information for you regarding using this food plan in the truck you can check it out here:

http://truckershealth.blogspot.com/

(check out 2012 post in the archive)

Conclusion

So by now your probably asking the question, "will this work for me?"

The answer is not simple due to the many factors involved in this disease. Personally I believe it will work for most people. I have talked to many people who have used this or a similar food plan who have had great success with reversing the course of this disease.

I have addressed primarily people whose disease can best be termed as Insulin Resistances Syndrome (I.R.S.).

Generally speaking I.R.S., is associated with being overweight and under-active. There are those with type 2 diabetes who are not over weight and under-active I have not spoke with many of them nor is it my experience with this disease. That being said, I think this food plan can help them but they should work closely with their doctor.

It is my belief that this disease is a nutrition problem. Our food supply is becoming less able to meet our bodies demands as our soils are being depleted of their nutrients faster than the soil can re-supply through natural means, especially with modern farming methods.

In researching material for this book I did run across some promising research which further reinforced my belief that this disease is a nutritional problem. It seems that when a certain portion of the small intestines is removed in a person or lab animal I.R.S. diabetes disappears.

Our small intestines is where the nutrients from our food is absorbed into the blood stream to be used by our body. These researchers think that this portion of the intestines is manufacturing an unknown substance that creates the condition of insulin resistance. What they seem to be missing is that that portion of the small intestines they are removing is the part that absorbs the simple sugars (sugar, and flour are simple sugars) from our food. Personally I think, that the typical American diet and our changing nutritional needs as we age is the real culprit.

Finally, try this food plan for three weeks and see if your blood sugar doesn't improve.

What do have to lose?

www.ingramcontent.com/pod-product-compliance
Lightning Source LLC
Chambersburg PA
CBHW071013180526
45168CB00003B/1410